Unlocking the Dementia Puzzle: A Revolutionary Guide to Cognitive Health and Empowered Living

By

NEVILLE LAWSON

Copyright © (NEVILLE LAWSON) 2023 All rights reserved

Before this document is duplicated or reproduced in any manner, the publisher's consent must be gained.

Table of contents

Preface

This is "Unlocking The Dementia Puzzle: A Revolutionary Guide to Cognitive Health and Empowered Living." We will introduce you to a layout of this book's items, objectives, and target readership in this context.

Introduction

A large number of individuals and their families are influenced by dementia, a worldwide well-being concern. It's a muddled problem that is habitually misdiagnosed and can essentially affect individuals' lives. This book is focused on uncovering the secrets of dementia and giving a careful outline of mental well-being, alongside guidance on the most proficient method to carry on with areas of strength for a full life despite mental issues.

The Book's Goal

This book fills two needs. Fundamentally, it intends to explain the intricacies of dementia and its different appearances, going from Alzheimer's illness to vascular dementia and then some. By revealing insight into the causes, signs, and course of dementia, we desire to dissipate a portion of the disgrace related to the sickness. We will likewise talk about momentum research on making due, treating ting, and forestalling dementia.

Second, we need to give helpful data and apparatuses to empower individuals with dementia and the people who care for them. A significant and useful life doesn't need to end due to dementia. We'll discuss how to keep your brain solid, improve your satisfaction, and make an emotionally supportive network that energizes versatility and strength.

Target Audience

Considering that dementia influences many individuals, this book is intended for an expansive crowd of perusers. Our fundamental gathering of interest comprises of:

1. People and Families: If you or a friend or family member has been determined to have dementia or is in danger, this book will give you significant data on the disease and supportive tips on changing the following mental issues.

2. Parental figures and Medical services Experts: This book is an extraordinary device for really focusing on people with dementia, assisting them with better figuring out dementia, fostering their providing care capacities, and keeping them informed about the latest improvements in the field.

3. Scientists and Understudies: This book offers broad experiences and references that will be

useful to analysts working in the field of mental well-being, understudies seeking medical care-related acts, and any other person keen on finding out about dementia.

4. For All Perusers: This book presents an unmistakable perspective on maturing, mental wellbeing, and getting a charge out of life without limit — regardless of whether you have no private involvement in dementia. For anyone with any interest at all in well-being and prosperity, it offers an extensive point of view on dementia.

I trust this book will be a useful aid for those exploring the much of the time puzzling and troublesome dementia venture. You'll have a superior comprehension of the dementia puzzle by the end, alongside the assets you want to carry on with a cheerful, free life. I'm thankful that you have gone along with me on this experience.

Chapter 1:

Does Dementia Exist?

At the point when an individual's ability to do every day errands is compromised, different mental disabilities are alluded to as dementia. It alludes to an assortment of side effects associated with a decrease in mental capability as opposed to a solitary disease. The side effects of dementia now and again create with time because the condition is habitually moderate. Cognitive decline, adjustments in language, thought, and thinking, as well as difficulties with critical thinking, are a few instances of these mental circumstances. A few basic clinical problems can prompt dementia, and the specific reason for the infection will decide how the side effects manifest.

classifications of dementia

1. Alzheimer's disease

As of now representing 60-70% of dementia cases, Alzheimer's illness is the most predominant reason for dementia. In the mind, variant protein stores, including tau tangles and beta-amyloid plaques, are gathering and causing a degenerative cerebral disease. Cognitive decline, disarray, and inconvenience of doing day-to-day assignments are brought about by these issues, which obstruct synapse correspondence. One's ability for correspondence and acknowledgment friends and family might be compromised as Alzheimer's advances.

2. Neurodegeneration or vascular dementia

There are two principal sorts of dementia: vascular and Alzheimer's. It comes from illnesses like strokes, little vessel infections, or other vascular issues that decrease blood supply to the cerebrum. Independent direction, arranging, and fixation issues are among the side effects of vascular dementia that could contrast as per the area and level of mind harm. Vascular dementia can progress in advance; side effects may not generally be obvious right away; they might settle for some time before declining once more.

3. Lewy Body Dementia

Unusual protein stores in the mind known as Lewy bodies are a sign of Lewy body dementia in patients. A few side effects of Parkinson's and Alzheimer's illnesses are shared by this sort of dementia. Visualizations, changes in the degree of mindfulness, and quakes are normal development side effects in individuals with Lewy body dementia. On account of its uncommon side effect mix, it very well may be hard to analyze and treat.

4. Frontotemporal Dementia

The cerebrum's front-facing and worldly curves are the primary regions impacted by frontotemporal dementia (FTD), a less pervasive type of dementia in general. Rather than being connected to cognitive decline, it is connected to modifications in conduct, character, and language. Phonological variety FTD, essential moderate aphasia, and semantic variation essential moderate aphasia are three unique ways that FTD can introduce itself, and they all have different side effect profiles.

5. Fascinating Dementia

At the point when somebody has different dementias simultaneously, ordinarily Alzheimer's sickness in addition to another sort, like vascular dementia, it's called blended dementia. A clinical appearance that is more perplexing can result from the blend of numerous pathologies.

6. Extra More uncommon Species

Wernicke-Korsakoff disorder, Huntington's sickness, and Creutzfeldt-Jakob illness are a couple of less common kinds of dementia notwithstanding the ones previously referenced. The side effects and hidden reasons for these ailments are particular.

Information and Pervasiveness

Dementia influences individuals all around the world and impacts families, medical care frameworks, and people. As far as the pervasiveness of dementia, a few significant pieces of information are:

In 2020, just about 50 million people overall were supposed to have dementia, as per the World Wellbeing Association (WHO). With the maturing populace being the primary element, this figure is supposed to almost quadruple by 2050, arriving at around 152 million. With an undeniably normal event, Alzheimer's sickness explicitly positions as the 6th most normal reason for mortality in the US.

Alongside the people beset, parental figures and the medical care framework are likewise troubled by dementia. The personal satisfaction of individuals with dementia and their families should be improved, and this requires expanding mindfulness, empowering early analysis, and carrying out proficient intercessions.

Chapter 2:

Dementia's Causes and Chance Elements

Dementia is a convoluted and various problem that can be caused or influenced by certain factors. Understanding these causes and hazard factors is basic for anticipation, early revelation, and successful administration. In this part, we will look all the more carefully at the essential drivers of dementia, like maturing, hereditary qualities, way of life factors, clinical issues, ecological effects, head wounds, and the job of hereditary qualities.

1. Aging and Hereditary qualities

Aging is the absolute most significant gambling factor for dementia. The gamble of having dementia ascends with age. This is because the mind changes normally over time, more inclined to mischief and illness. Hereditary qualities likewise play a significant effect in the possibility of getting dementia. Family ancestry can be a major area of strength for a singular's helplessness to specific types of dementia, like Alzheimer's illness. Even though they are exceptional, a few hereditary changes have been connected to an expanded gamble of dementia.

2. Lifestyle Elements

A singular's way of life decisions can essentially affect their possibility of getting dementia. Unfortunate propensities like unfortunate food, absence of active work, smoking, unreasonable liquor consumption, and ongoing pressure can all raise the gamble. A solid way of life, then again, including a decent eating routine, incessant work-out, mental feeling, and social commitment, can assist with bringing down the gamble of dementia.

3. Ailments

Certain clinical issues can raise the gamble of dementia. Hypertension, diabetes, and elevated cholesterol, for instance, have all been connected to an expanded gamble of dementia. Stoutness and rest issues may likewise add to mental crumbling. Viable administration of these clinical problems can limit the gamble of dementia.

4. Natural Elements

Natural factors like air contamination, harmful openness, and a lack of admittance to schooling and medical care can all add to the improvement of dementia. Drawing out openness to hazardous substances or living in a contaminated climate might have unfortunate results on mind well-being. Besides, limited admittance to quality medical services and schooling could bring about botched open doors for early intercession and counteraction.

5. Head Wounds

Head injuries, especially horrendous mind wounds (TBIs), are a realized gamble factor for dementia. A solid hit to the head, as may happen in mishaps or sports-related wounds, can cause long-term mental harm and raise the gamble of mental degradation and dementia. Preventive systems and cautious administration of head wounds are basic in bringing down this gamble.

6. The Capability of Hereditary Qualities

Hereditary qualities play a mind-boggling part in the improvement of dementia. While most instances of dementia are not straightforwardly acquired, certain hereditary variables can raise weakness to explicit types of dementia. For instance, the APOE 4 quality has been connected to an expanded gamble of Alzheimer's sickness. Understanding one's hereditary affinity can assist with settling on informed choices concerning their way of life and medical services.

7. Perceiving Hazard Variables

Perceiving the gamble factors for dementia is basic for early mediation and counteraction. Medical care experts, as well as patients and their families, ought to be taught about these gambling factors. Ordinary mental tests and well-being screenings can assist with distinguishing early signs of mental crumbling, taking into consideration proper intercessions to bring down the gamble and successfully oversee dementia.

In the accompanying parts, we will take a gander at dementia conclusion, treatment, and care options, extending in light of data made here about its causes and hazard factors.

Chapter 3:

Cerebrum Capability and Dementia

To get a handle on the mental modifications experienced by dementia patients, one priority is an exhaustive comprehension of the perplexing communication between dementia and the cerebrum. The construction and capability of the mind, how it changes in dementia, crafted by synapses, and the utilization of neuroimaging in dementia findings are completely shrouded in this section.

1. Design and Capability of the Brain

Our whole scope of feelings, ways of behaving, and considerations are administered by the amazingly multifaceted human mind. It is partitioned into a few regions, every one of which plays out a specific job. For instance, the transient curve is engaged with language and memory, the cerebrum administers independent direction and character, and the hippocampus is fundamental for the production of new recollections.

2. Dementia-Related Brain Modifications

Moderate and broad brain decay, essentially influencing mental capability, is a sign of dementia. The development of deviant protein stores (like tau and beta-amyloid) and the deficiency of neurons and neurotransmitters are normal mind irregularities related to dementia. Memory, rationale, language, and other mental capabilities might endure because of these modifications.

3. Synapses' job

Synthetic compounds called synapses are liable for signal transmission in the mind, which empowers neuronal correspondence. Synapse lopsided characteristics can altogether influence the mind's capabilities. Certain synapses, similar to acetylcholine, which is fundamental for memory and learning, are found in lower focuses in dementia, particularly Alzheimer's illness. Mental decay is exacerbated by this compound unevenness.

4. Diagnosing dementia with neuroimaging

The determination and cognizance of dementia are enormously supported by neuroimaging strategies. They work with the perception of the life systems and capability of the mind by clinical subject matter experts, supporting the discovery of oddities. While diagnosing dementia, normal neuroimaging procedures include:

An attractive reverberation imaging (X-ray) filters a careful picture of the cerebrum's life systems by X-ray, which makes it possible to recognize dementia-related irregularities like injuries, decay, and different changes.

Registered tomography, or CT examines, and identifies physical anomalies in the cerebrum, for example, cancers or harmed locales, which might be connected to dementia.

- PET (Positron Outflow Tomography) filters: These imaging strategies underscore specific cerebrum problems and capabilities by utilizing radioactive tracers. modifications in glucose digestion are regularly recognized by them, and these changes might be an indication of dementia.

- **SPECT (Single Photon Discharge Processed Tomography) checks:** These outputs survey the cerebral bloodstream and help in the finding of different dementias.

To precisely analyze and order dementia and empower the clinical workforce to offer the right consideration and backing, neuroimaging procedures are utilized related to clinical appraisals and mental testing.

Expanding on the essential data introduced in this section about the mind's part in dementia, we will investigate the different types of dementia in more detail in the accompanying parts, alongside their clinical attributes and potential medicines.

Chapter 4:

Diagnosis of Dementia

The conclusion of dementia is a fundamental stage in the administration and care of those impacted by this problem. In this section, we will take a gander at the early advance notice side effects of dementia, the demonstrative cycle, mental evaluation, clinical trials, and the significance of early location.

1. Early Admonition Signs

Perceiving the early admonition indications of dementia is basic for suitable finding and intercession. These signs might include:

- Memory issues: Continuous neglecting, particularly for ongoing occasions or fundamental subtleties.

- Trouble with errands: Attempting to do everyday errands like cooking or overseeing funds.
- Language challenges: trouble tracking down words, clarifying expressions, or following conversations.
- Bewilderment: Becoming mixed up in recognizable areas, forgetting about time, or feeling confused.
- Misguided thinking: Going with sketchy choices, prominently ones that imperil security.
- Mind-set and character change: Displaying quick emotional episodes, character changes, or social detachment.
- Mental degradation: diminished critical abilities to think, restricted theoretical reasoning, and more unfortunate thinking.

2. The Indicative Technique

Dementia finding is a convoluted cycle that typically contains a few stages:

- Clinical History: Medical services experts accumulate data concerning the patient's clinical history, including any family background of dementia.

- Physical and neurological assessment
An actual assessment distinguishes plausible basic clinical issues, though a neurological evaluation assesses mental and engine execution.

- **Mental Evaluation**: Mental tests and polls, like the Small Mental State Assessment (MMSE), are utilized to survey memory, consideration, language, and other mental regions.

- **Clinical trials**: Clinical trials are utilized to preclude different diseases that could be causing the noticed side effects. These may incorporate blood testing, imaging assessments (X-ray, CT, PET), and cerebrospinal liquid investigation.

3. Mental Assessment

Mental testing is a significant piece of the dementia-indicative strategy. Different state-administered tests and polls are utilized to survey mental capability, memory, and critical thinking skills. These assessments give medical services suppliers helpful bits of knowledge into the level and nature of mental weakness, aiding the separation of dementia from different diseases that might give comparative side effects.

4. Clinical Tests

Clinical trials are basic in the analytic stage since they assist with precluding other potential reasons for mental impedance. A few normal clinical trials are:

- Blood tests: These can identify or preclude diseases like lack of nutrients, thyroid issues, and contaminants that can debilitate memory.

- Imaging studies: X-ray, CT outputs, and PET sweeps give nitty gritty pictures of the mind, aiding the recognizable proof of primary irregularities or changes in cerebrum capability.

- Cerebrospinal fluid examination: A lumbar cut can be utilized to read up cerebrospinal liquid for indications of certain sorts of dementia, like Alzheimer's sickness.

5. The Significance of Early Conclusion

Early dementia conclusion is basic in light of multiple factors:

- Early intercession: Distinguishing dementia in its beginning phases considers prompt clinical and social mediations, which can help with easing back the movement of the illness and upgrade the singular's satisfaction.

- Treatment and backing: Early analysis permits medical services suppliers to give fitting therapy, backing, and instruction to both the person with dementia and their guardians.

- Future preparation: Early conclusion assists families with planning for the future, making lawful and monetary courses of action, and guaranteeing that the individual with dementia gets the most ideal thought that anybody could expect to find.

- Clinical preliminary interest: Early conclusion grants support in clinical preliminaries and exploration studies, which are urgent for encouraging comprehension. We might interpret dementia and find new treatments.

In the accompanying parts, we will look at treatment decisions as well as procedures for giving consideration and backing to individuals with dementia and their families, expanding on the information introduced in this section about dementia conclusion.

Chapter 5:

Guidelines to Manage a Dementia Diagnosis

Both the person with dementia and their loved ones could see getting a dementia finding as an irksome and significant event. The up close and personal expense that a dementia end can have, correspondence methodologies, the value of empowering gatherings, future readiness, and significant genuine and money-related issues will be covered in this part.

1. Significant Effect

A dementia assurance could make one experience wonderment, fear, pity, or anxiety, among other feelings. As they fight with the movements dementia will bring to their lives, people could experience a sensation of mishap.

A critical piece of the cycle is sorting out some way to manage these feelings.

2. Presenting the Condition

It might be a fragile and irksome cycle to decide if someone has dementia. Specialists in the clinical benefits industry ought to convey this in an open, certifiable, and caring way. This figures out the kind of dementia, the way things are made, and such prescriptions that are available. Open and enabling correspondence among relatives is comparably basic.

3. System Support

For those with dementia and individuals who care for them, having serious areas of strength for a gathering is central. Family, partners, empowering gatherings, and clinical specialists could be all around a piece of this system. In particular, support packs provide a safeguarded environment for people to share their records, get obliging headings, and get essential consolation.

4. Forward-Looking Course of action

One of the essential bits of dealing with a dementia finding is making arrangements. Picking between extended-length thought, abiding, and clinical ideas is huge for this cycle. A singular's objectives are respected whether or not they can't seek decisions for themselves in light of advance thought orchestrating, which consolidates making advance requests and allotting an overall legitimate expert for clinical consideration.

5. A Look at the Law and Resources

Following a finding of dementia, managing lawful and monetary issues is basic:

- Legal approaches: These incorporate earning enough to pay the bills will or propelling clinical consideration command, assigning a strong legitimate expert for assets, and setting up a will. To guarantee the genuine adequacy of these reports, legitimate guidance could be required.

- Financial arrangement: Dementia's money-related effects ought to be surveyed. Families and individuals should examine Bureaucratic clinical protection and Medicaid decisions, long-stretch consideration assurance, and their capability for government help programs.

- Inheritance organizing: This includes picking how to course a single asset after their passing. This could incorporate setting up trusts, completely taking into account the obligation suggestions, and being properly named to guarantee the beneficiaries.

Getting dementia assurance is a long communication that requires hard work and understanding to be investigated. Family members and parental figures ought to zero in on their own significant and close-to-home prosperity to offer their loved ones with dementia the best possible assistance.

Chapter 6:

Treatment and The management

Viable dementia treatment and management require a complex methodology that consolidates drugs, treatments, way-of-life changes, and non-pharmacological medications. This part digs into these issues, including prescription administration challenges and the possibility of clinical preliminaries and exploratory medicines.

1. Prescriptions and Treatments

There are different medications and treatments utilized in the treatment and the executives of dementia, especially for explicit structures like Alzheimer's sickness:

 - **Cholinesterase inhibitors**: Cholinesterase inhibitors, like Donepezil, Rivastigmine, and

Galantamine, are habitually controlled to work on mental execution and decrease a portion of the side effects related to Alzheimer's illness.

- NMDA receptor adversaries: Memantine is an NMDA receptor bad guy used to get moderate extreme Alzheimer's infection side effects, especially those connected to memory and mental capability.

- Conduct and mental treatment: These treatments attempt to oversee risky ways of behaving and further develop the general prosperity of individuals with dementia. Mental social treatment, reality direction, and memory treatment are a few medicines used to treat mental and close-to-home problems.

2. Non-pharmacological Intercessions

Non-pharmacological treatments are basic in dementia treatment. These are a few models:

- Mental feeling: Exercises that animate mental abilities, for example, puzzles, memory games, and imaginative endeavors can help with holding mental capacities.

- Active work: Customary activity works on both physical and psychological wellness. It can help mindset, bring down the gamble of cardiovascular infection, and work on mental execution.

- Dietary intercessions: A fair eating routine wealthy in cell reinforcements and Omega-3 unsaturated fats might keep up with mind capability and limit the gamble of mental degradation.

- Tangible methodologies, like music treatment and fragrant healing, can bring close-to-home solace and invigorate memory review.

3. Way of life Alterations

Way of life changes are significant in dementia the board:

-Diet: A solid eating routine rich in cell reinforcements is remembered to help mind wellbeing. Sugar and soaked fat decrease is likewise encouraged.

- Work out. Ordinary actual work can upgrade cardiovascular well-being, lessen pressure, and lift general prosperity.

- Mental excitement: Taking part in mentally animating exercises like perusing, riddles, and acquiring new abilities can help with supporting mental capability.

- Social commitment: Keeping up with connections and remaining socially dynamic are basic for close-to-home and mental well-being.

4. Clinical Preliminaries and Exploratory Medicines

Clinical preliminaries and exploratory medicines are opportunities for researching new strategies for dementia on the board. These investigations take a gander at planned medications, treatments, and intercessions to assist individuals with dementia in carrying on with better lives. Cooperation in clinical preliminaries can give admittance to state-of-the-art medicines while likewise adding to the improvement of dementia research.

5. Medicine Organization Troubles

Medicine organization in dementia care can be troublesome, particularly as the condition progresses. Normal challenges include:

- Prescription adherence: Dementia patients might neglect to take their remedies or may decline to take them attributable to mental or conduct issues.

- Polypharmacy: Dealing with various medications, each with its portion plan, can be troublesome. Drug systems should be smoothed out whenever the situation allows.

- Medicine incidental effects: Some dementia medications might have side impacts, which should be painstakingly checked and made due.

- Prescription associations: People with dementia might be taking numerous meds for different medical problems, making it basic to be aware of potential medication corporations.

Treatment and the executives' choices ought to be custom-fitted to the singular's requirements and conditions. Ordinary conversations with medical services experts and parental figures are expected to evaluate therapy viability and make essential adjustments.

In the accompanying parts, we will take a gander at the difficulties of providing care, techniques for working on the personal satisfaction of individuals with dementia, and the moral and legitimate issues that accompany dementia care, expanding on the fundamental information given in this section about treatment and management.

Chapter 7:

Giving care to Patients with Dementia

Relatives and other direct relations now and again take on the troublesome and huge assignment of really focusing on individuals who have dementia. The job of guardians is analyzed in this part, alongside survival techniques for parental figure pressure, care group arrangement, acquiring support administrations and relief care, and security and house enhancements.

1. The guardians' job

In the existence of those enduring dementia, guardians are significant. Their arrangement of common sense, profound, and actual help supports safeguarding their friends and family's well-being and way of life. Parental figures offer help with ordinary undertakings, regulate medication organization, and lay out a solid and steady air.

2. Overseeing Pressure for Guardians

It may very well be genuinely and depleting to focus on somebody who has dementia. Stress among guardians is far and wide and can take many structures, including burnout, nervousness, misery, and medical conditions. Among the methods to oversee parental figure pressure are:

Self-care: Keeping up with physical and emotional well-being requires taking care of oneself — through normal activity, a sound eating regimen, and enough rest — need.

- Encouraging groups of people: Looking for help from loved ones and joining support gatherings can assist with reducing the close-to-home kind of giving consideration.

  - Relief care: Administrations for parental figures that proposition transient alleviation so they can unwind and restore.

3. Shaping an Assenting Gathering

A consideration group, which can incorporate relatives, local area assets, and clinical specialists, is much of the time more viable while giving consideration. Giving exhaustive consideration requires colleagues to team up and discuss well with each other.

4. Backing and Reprieve Care Administrations

Transitory alleviation for parental figures is given by relief care. This is accessible in various arrangements:

  - In-home reprieve: Support for parental figures can be given at home by volunteers or qualified experts.

Programs for those with dementia that give administered care during the day let loose guardians to deal with themselves.

- Transient private consideration: Relief care can be given for expanded time frames at foundations like helped residing networks or nursing homes.

To assist parental figures with dealing with their commitments, support administrations including advice, monetary and lawful direction, and training about dementia can be exceptionally useful.

5. Security and Transformations to the Home

It is imperative to safeguard the prosperity of those experiencing dementia. Among the progressions to a house are:

- Fall avoidance: The risk of falls can be diminished by eliminating trip dangers, adding get bars, and ensuring there is adequate light.

- **Meandering counteraction**: You can assist with holding individuals with dementia back from wandering and getting derailed by introducing entryway cautions, locks, and customized IDs.

- Medicine the executives: Prescription coordinators or clear names can assist with guaranteeing the right organization, and drugs ought to be put away in a safe area.

- Memory helps: Update frameworks or marking cupboards and drawers can assist individuals with dementia in dealing with their environmental elements.

To lay out a protected and empowering home climate, guardians ought to perform routine well-being assessments and make changes as needed.

While considering an individual experiencing dementia can be sincerely satisfying, there are sure troubles included. Viable care requires conveying treatment, searching for help, and setting up well-being precautionary measures. To ensure the best personal satisfaction for every interested individual, the carer's and the dementia patient's requirements ought to start things out.

Chapter 8:

Overseeing Dementia

Both the people who have dementia and the individuals who care for them have specific issues while living with the disease. This section takes a gander at different points, incorporating conquering impediments in everyday living, imparting, and safeguarding one's freedom, setting up a dementia-accommodating climate, and working on the overall personal satisfaction of dementia patients.

1. Snags in Day to day existence

An individual with dementia might confront various snags in their day-to-day existence, for example,

Recollecting names, countenances, and ongoing occasions is quite difficult for individuals experiencing dementia.

- Correspondence: It can turn out to be increasingly more challenging to figure out others and to offer your viewpoints.

- Simply deciding: Going with choices can get overwhelming, in any event, concerning necessities like garments or food.

Safety: Individuals experiencing dementia might be inclined to meander, fall, or disregard their eating routine and individual cleanliness.

To conquer these deterrents and advance the individual's prosperity, parental figures need to alter their methodology.

2. Techniques for Correspondence

Both the people who are focusing on somebody with dementia and the actual individual need to successfully impart. Procedures comprise of:

- Work on language: To work on understanding, use language that is clear, compact, and direct.

- Undivided attention: Give the individual space to painstakingly talk and pay attention to them.

- Non-verbal signs: See how individuals move their body, make looks, and talk.

- Approval and redirection: Regard the individual's feelings, regardless of whether what they say isn't correct. Moving the discussion to a more perky subject could diminish strain.

3. Supporting Uniqueness

Individuals with dementia must keep up with their feelings of freedom. To do this, a few methodologies are as per the following:

- Improve on work by partitioning day-to-day tasks into little, attainable advances.

Advance association by affecting the individual in navigation and exercises that are fitting for their ability level.

- Versatile hardware: Use gear, like marks or updates for routine errands, to help free living.

Laying out a Setting That Is Dementia-Accommodating

For those experiencing dementia, creating changes to their living space can improve their satisfaction. This incorporates:

Protected and available plan: Dispose of deterrents, ensure ways are self-evident, and adjust the house to fit those with restricted versatility.

- Obvious signs: Simplify it for individuals to explore their current circumstances by utilizing marks, signs, and a variety of coding.

Schedules, whiteboards, and marked drawers are instances of memory help that can be utilized to help individuals review obligations and schedules.

5. Further developing Future

Working on the personal satisfaction for the people who have dementia involves:

Cooperation in significant exercises: Advance your quest for advantages, interests, and pursuits that make you cheerful and provide you with a feeling of progress.

- Social connection: To decrease sensations of forlornness, keep in contact with loved ones.

- mental and actual excitement: Mental undertakings, tactile encounters, and standard activity can all add to general prosperity.

At the point when these methods are applied to improve an individual's satisfaction, considering somebody who has dementia can genuinely be satisfied. It's basic to remember that individuals experiencing dementia can in any case be cheerful, associate with their current circumstance, and have satisfying connections.

The following parts will address end-of-life arrangements, moral and legitimate issues in dementia care, and different assets that can be utilized to work on the personal satisfaction of both dementia patients and their carers. This material develops the experiences introduced in this part concerning maturing with dementia.

Chapter 9:

Lawful and Moral Issues

Legitimate and moral contemplations are basic pieces of dementia care, particularly as the condition propels. This section plunges into advanced mandates, guardianship and conservatorship, moral issues in dementia care, end-of-life navigation, and the capability of a senior regulation lawyer.

1. Advance Orders

Advance orders are legitimate arrangements that permit people to characterize their clinical treatment inclinations and choose a medical services intermediary to settle on choices for their benefit when they are as of now not ready to do so. Advance mandates can detail people with dementia's cravings for worries like life-supporting treatments, revival, and hospice care.

- Living Will: A living will frames an individual's desires for clinical medicines, especially end-of-life care.

- Strong Legal authority for Medical care: This record chooses a reliable person to settle on medical care decisions for the benefit of the person with dementia when they can't do so themselves.

Advance orders are basic for guaranteeing that a singular's desires are regarded in any event, when they can't express them.

2. Guardianship and Conservatorship

People experiencing dementia might become incapable of going with their own choices, especially those unsettling their monetary worries, as the sickness advances. In such occasions, guardianship or conservatorship might be required. These legitimate courses of action select somebody to pursue decisions for the individual with dementia.

   - Guardianship: A gatekeeper is typically responsible for settling on private and clinical decisions for the person.

   - Conservatorship: A conservator deals with a person's monetary and legitimate undertakings.

These legitimate activities ought to be looked for where there is an evident need to shield the individual with dementia and deal with their undertakings to their greatest advantage.

3. Moral Contemplations

In dementia care, moral contemplations outweigh everything else. Guardians and medical care experts should fight moral problems, for example,

   - Adjusting independence and security: It may very well be challenging to regard a singular's independence while safeguarding their security, particularly when they take part in dangerous situations.

- Trustworthiness: Choosing whether to uncover a dementia determination in the impacted individual is a troublesome moral issue. Trustworthiness should be adjusted against the potential for trouble.

- End-of-life care: Moral choices about finish-of-life care, including the withdrawal of life-supporting medicines, ought to be directed by the singular's desires and well-being.

4. Pursuing Finish of-Life Choices

End-of-life choices are critical for individuals experiencing progressed dementia. These choices might incorporate the utilization of advanced mandates, like living wills, to administer medical care choices. End-of-life care morals ought to focus on the singular's solace, pride, and personal satisfaction.

5. The Job of a Senior Regulation Lawyer

Senior regulation lawyers have some expertise in legitimate difficulties influencing more seasoned grown-ups, quite those experiencing dementia. Their job in dementia care might include:

- Helping with advance mandates: A senior regulation lawyer can help create and execute advance orders, guaranteeing they consent to state guidelines.

- Guardianship and conservatorship: At the point when fundamental, lawyers can help families explore the legitimate course of securing guardianship or conservatorship.

- Bequest arranging: Senior regulation experts can help people with dementia and their families in setting up their monetary and legitimate undertakings, like wills, trusts, and Medicaid arranging.

A senior regulation lawyer's experience can be urgent in exploring the complex legitimate scene of dementia care.

Chapter 10:

Neighborhood Assets and Help

For the people who are focusing on somebody with dementia, approaching local area assets and help is essential. This part looks at various administrations and assets that can direct individuals through the hardships of really focusing on a friend or family member with dementia and assisting them with finding the help they require.

1. Affiliations and Associations for Dementia

Data, promotion, and backing are significantly helped by dementia social orders and associations. These associations now and again center around expanding consciousness of dementia and upgrading the existence of the individuals who are influenced by it. Among the notable organizations are:

- Alzheimer's Affiliation: This gathering fund-raises for research on Alzheimer's illness and gives instructive materials and backing administrations.

- The Lewy Body Dementia Affiliation: This association offers instructive assets and examination refreshes while focusing on helping individuals with Lewy body dementia and the people who care for them.

- Frontotemporal Lobar Degeneration Affiliation: Through examination, backing, and instruction, this association expects to help frontotemporal degeneration victims and their families.

2. Help Groups

Support bunches permit dementia patients and their carers a discussion to discuss their encounters, clarify pressing issues, and get consistent encouragement from individuals who know about the troubles they face. Various disconnected and online care groups center around specific types of dementia and give a solid climate to correspondence and training.

3. Programs for Rest Care

Programs for rest care give guardians transient relief so they can have some time off from their providing care obligations. These projects, which offer proficient consideration for individuals with dementia for a foreordained measure of time at home or in an office, permit guardians to enjoy some time off and refuel.

4. Therapy clinics for Memory

Offices for memory care are made to explicitly take care of the requirements of individuals who have dementia. They furnish a protected and empowering environment with laborers who have gotten particular dementia care preparation. Memory care foundations offer day programs or private consideration because of the requirements of the individual and the desires of the family.

5. Monetary help and government help

Monetary guides and government support projects can help families and people experiencing dementia in gathering the costs of their consideration. Contingent upon the region, these projects can include:

Medicaid: A joint government state program that offers low-pay individuals well-being inclusion, including long-haul care administrations.

Benefits from the Veterans Organization (VA): The VA offers types of assistance and advantages to veterans, including help for diseases like dementia that are connected with their tactical assistance.

- Government-managed retirement Handicap Protection (SSDI): SSDI offers monetary help to individuals who can't fill in because of a handicap, like dementia.

Monetary guides and government help projects might be difficult to reach specific people because of their pay, assets, and military assistance records.

People with dementia and their parental figures can track down priceless help and data to help them on their way by using these local area assets and backing administrations. These apparatuses can work on the personal satisfaction of dementia patients and ensure they get the help and care they need.

Chapter 11:

Future Headings and Exploration

Dementia research is basic to encouraging comprehension. We might interpret the problem and make novel ways to deal with avoidance and treatment. This part dives into proceeding with dementia research, possible disclosures, overall coordinated efforts, the chase after a fix, and the moral contemplations that underlie this basic area of study.

1. Progressing Dementia Exploration

Dementia research is a continually developing field with various momentum studies and investigations. Scientists investigate various themes, including:

- Biomarkers: Recognizing explicit natural pointers in the mind or blood that might help with early conclusion or ailment advancement.

- Hereditary qualities: Examining the hereditary factors that lead to different kinds of dementia, like Alzheimer's sickness.

- Treatment draws near Making and testing new medications, treatments, and intercessions to postpone the movement of dementia and work on mental capability.

- Risk factors: Researching way of life, ecological, and hereditary variables to all the more likely comprehend how they add to the improvement of dementia.

2. Possible Leap forwards

A few forthcoming progressions in dementia research have shown guarantee, including:

- Immunotherapies: Research examines safe-based prescriptions that target proteins connected to dementia, like beta-amyloid and tau.

- Early location devices: The production of additional precise and open strategies for early conclusion, which can further develop treatment adequacy.

- Customized medication: Fitting medicines to the unmistakable hereditary, biochemical, and mental attributes of dementia patients.

3. Worldwide Joint efforts

Cooperation in dementia research crosses public limits. Worldwide coordinated efforts empower analysts to share their disclosures, assets, and abilities. These exercises support common sense and speed progress in figuring out dementia and expected treatments.

4. The Chase after a Fix

The quest for a fix remains a high concentration in dementia research. While there is as of now no treatment for most assortments of dementia, specialists are proceeding to explore numerous conceivable outcomes, going from drug improvement to regenerative treatment. A definitive objective is to find intercessions that can forestall, slow, or invert the mental misfortune related to dementia.

5. Moral Contemplations in Dementia Exploration

Since dementia research includes weak people, moral contemplations are urgent. Key moral standards include:

- Informed assent: Guaranteeing those members partaking in research grasp the review's goal, likely dangers, and advantages.

- Member security: Safeguarding the privileges and prosperity of people with dementia, especially the individuals who might come up short on the ability to give informed assent.

- Straightforwardness: Guaranteeing that examination discoveries are passed openly on to people in general, medical care experts, and policymakers.

Moral issues are basic in dementia research to safeguard the nobility and privileges of people partaking in examinations and to keep up with public confidence in established researchers.

Dementia research is a dynamic and extending point that holds a colossal commitment to working on the existences of those impacted by the problem. Progressing studies and overall coordinated efforts are setting the street for likely forward leaps, and specialists are striving to acquire more profound information on dementia and, in the end, a fix.

Chapter 12:

Dementia- Accommodating Climate

Guaranteeing the nobility and prosperity of individuals with dementia requires the improvement of a general public that is dementia-accommodating. The various features of making a dementia-accommodating society are investigated in this part, including backing and regulative change, dementia-accommodating projects, bringing down disgrace, expanding mindfulness, and the worth of inclusivity.

1. Expanding Soul

The most important phase in making a general public that is dementia-accommodating is expanding public information on dementia. The effect of dementia and the challenges faced by the individuals who care for the people who have it tend to be better perceived by networks through open mindfulness crusades, instructive drives, and media drives. More noteworthy sympathy and understanding can result from expanded mindfulness.

2. Relieving Disgrace

Backing and care for those with dementia are seriously hampered by disgrace. To lessen disgrace, deceptions and ominous insights concerning dementia should be scattered. A comprehensive and sympathetic disposition toward people experiencing dementia can be encouraged and insights can be modified with the guidance of training and firsthand records.

3. Projects Amicable to Dementia

The objective of dementia-accommodating projects is to expand the openness and convenience of public regions and networks for individuals who have dementia. Among these drives could be:

- Dementia-accommodating organizations: Advancing the preparation of workers to be more thoughtful and sympathetic toward clients experiencing dementia.

- Networks that are dementia-accommodating: These areas could give safe regions for individuals with dementia to mingle, public travel that is open, and different conveniences.

- Memory bistros: These informal parties permit individuals with dementia and their carers to open doors in a soothing setting.

4. How Significant Inclusivity Is

The underpinning of a general public that is dementia-accommodating is inclusivity. This involves ensuring that individuals experiencing dementia get aware treatment and impartial admittance to assets and amazing open doors. By empowering a sensation of local area and social union, comprehensive practices help the individuals who are impacted by dementia as well as society at large.

5. Campaigning and Changing Approach

A dementia-accommodating society should be laid out through support and regulative changes. Crusade drives might comprise of:

- Initiating better admittance to dementia analysis, care, and treatment through campaigning for further developed medical care administrations.

Energize the creation and utilization of regulations that shield the freedoms and government assistance of individuals experiencing dementia to help regulation.

- Empowering examination and financing: Pushing for more cash to be designated to concentrate on that will assist us with grasping dementia and making pragmatic medicines.

Neighborhood, local, and public backing drives can support the execution of arrangements that improve the existence of dementia patients and their carers.

It requires collaboration with the dynamic contribution of people, networks, states, and associations to make a general public that is dementia-accommodating. We can assist in making an inviting and steady air for people with dementia by expanding mindfulness, bringing down disgrace, and pushing for change.

Chapter 13:

Individual Encounters and Stories

In the setting of dementia, individual stories and encounters can give essential bits of knowledge and motivation. We will take a gander at first-individual records, guardian tributes, medical services proficient perceptions, and moving instances of adapting and versatility in this section, all of which illuminate the lived encounters of individuals with dementia and the people who care for them.

1. Individual Records

First-individual stories give extraordinary knowledge into the regular routines and issues of those living with dementia. These accounts much of the time portray the feelings, difficulties, and triumphs of people influenced by the sickness. They refine the experience and present a more complete image of what it's preferred to live with dementia.

2. Tributes from Guardians

Guardian tributes give knowledge about the commitments, delights, and difficulties that the individuals who care for individuals with dementia experience. These accounts underline the personal ties that guardians structure with their friends and family, as well as the penances and commitment that providing care requires.

3. Medical services Experts' Points of view

Medical services staff who work with dementia patients can give fundamental knowledge about the condition. Their points of view on the clinical and profound parts of dementia care, as well as the creating field of dementia examination and treatment, are adjusted.

4. Moving Adapting and Strength Stories

There are various accounts of ingenuity, relentlessness, and the human soul's capacity to drive forward through the difficulties of dementia. These moving stories feature the phenomenal achievements and variations of individuals living with dementia, as well as the dedication and fondness of guardians.

Individual stories and encounters help to instruct, spur, and interface individuals from the dementia local area. They can carry comfort to people confronting comparable troubles and critical examples to guardians and medical services experts.

Unlocking the dementia puzzle.

I HOPE YOU GOT VALUE.....?

THE END

9 798865 939696